Blissful Living

*A Guide to
Transform your
Life Now*

LENA PREMLEENA WETTERGRAN

Ordering Information:

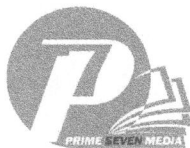

Prime Seven Media
518 Landmann St.
Tomah City, WI 54660

Printed in the United States of America

Table of Contents

Foreword

This might sound like a bad script. I was at the peak of my career; I had a family. I was running a successful business. But I was completely broken within me, and I wanted to escape it all. I was wandering through a park in Stockholm one day, despondent and alone, it seemed. I looked up to see an old friend standing there. He was gravely concerned by my appearance. I told him I was not well and that I would probably take a trip to Barcelona to get away from everything. He looked at me for a moment and then suggested that I go somewhere else. In hindsight, this seems orchestrated, like an intervention from above that was clandestine.

That weekend I put the keys into my car's ignition and raced through the countryside. Something seemed to be propelling me forward. I was overdressed and I was late. I looked like an asshole of the highest order. I thought I should probably turn around and forget this ever happened. But still, there was something inexplicably pulling me forward. Eventually, I found myself at a door, so I opened that door. Then I found myself at a set of stairs, so I walked up those stairs. Then I was greeted by a woman, so I apologized. She told me they were waiting. I was on time and everything was perfect.

There were people sitting quietly on the floor in meditation chairs and a woman beaming in the centre. She warmly welcomed me. She was both ageless and timeless, almost like a teenager, with a wild heart and playful energy like a child. I sat down and I listened. It became clear to me that she would require only one thing. I had to leave everything behind, my expectations, persona, ideas, success and ego. In those initial moments, I realized that this was the beginning of a journey that would slowly guide me back home toward myself. Her name is Premleena, Lena Wettergran and she changed my life. Since that first encounter 20 years ago, she has taught me so much about myself and my wounding.

Now, you have this book in your hands, a concentrated version of what I have learned from her during all the years and still is.. I am giving the keys to you. But what you may not realize is that you have already opened the door by reading this. The tools in this book will bring you to aspects of yourself that you might rather keep hidden. However, if you embrace these teachings you may come to an understanding like I did. I was able to unlock creativity, loving me, my family more deeply, understand leadership and approach my work fearlessly.

I am a creative businessman, but I am not complicated when it comes to my approach. Similarly, this program is concrete, adaptable; nothing fancy. I believe that no matter who you are, this book can help you come into your highest, most authentic self. Whether it is finding success or love, these core principles will filter into every aspect of your journey. I'm not a religious man, but I believe that being open is the only way forward. This book will help you finding your own truth, My advice to you would be: stay present and let go. I wish you the best on your journey – and be kind to yourself.

Ps. Off course it is a big difference from reading truth and get guidance in a book, from experience first hand, for your self in group processes with Premleena. So if you have a chance to meet her that way, to get the guidance that way, I highly recommend that.

Peter Settman

Entrepreneur and TV Producer

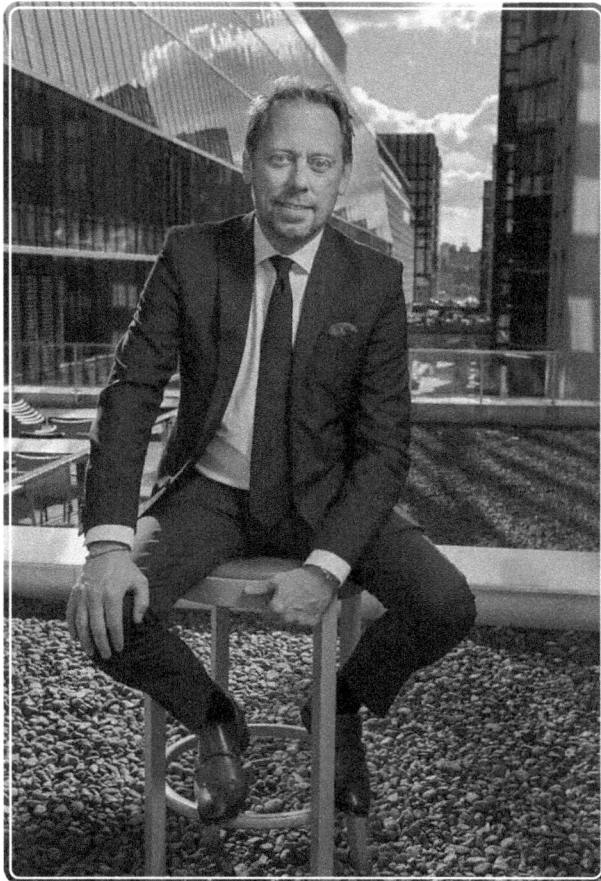

Introduction

I wish this book to be like luke warm running water on to ice, melting it. Melting all that stand between you are your authentic divine self. Your greatest adventure, to turn within and meet your own inner self. Ready to walk our own truth.

In this book, I am going to guide you on how to bring peace, abundance, and bliss into your life, to embrace who you really are with bringing awareness.

True health and wealth is the outcome of knowing oneself, to find our inner leadership. Bliss is an invitation to start living your own inner truth; it's freedom in true abundance.

Blissful living…

is for me when we turn within, to live in connection and trust, beyond the mind's stressful chatter, connected with our hearts and love, as with the graceful essence we are, knowing that all is interconnected and that we are all a perfect part of this magical universe.

True abundance…

is for me to be alive, trusting, flowering and receiving life as it is.

… trusting my own inner graceful self… where health and wealth go together in perfect harmony.

Transformation

Change is natural and to move into higher forms of consciousness is natural… being this energy, alive and allowing. Moving to our hearts and transformation starts to happen.

Like a butterfly coming out of its chrysalis,

Like a flower coming out of its bud into full flowering.

Trust this ever-changing existence and its ever silent wisdom. Welcome home, beloved. Meeting yourself is the greatest gift of all.

My own experience and transforming life process:

Seven doors to awakening, all equally important in Self leadership, all-dancing together, this I call blissful living.

Chapter 1

The invitation, stop running away!

There is nowhere to go… high time to come home.
Connect within, finding what you are longing
for… life as an awakening process …

Chapter 2

The bigger picture!

We are pure universal consciousness in human form,
so much more than we ever think or believe.
When we become aware that we all are
connected, it all becomes possible.

Chapter 3

Emotional healing, clearing the past!

To free yourself, stepping beyond mind and the old… master your
life with a healthy mind and open heart… finding your truth.

Chapter 4

To be the radiance of the love you truly are!

Trusting your own heart… Loving yourself, your partner and
others. To value presence in endless bliss and abundance.

Chapter 5

Living in a yes!

Being the central person in your own life … you are
already here, in the river of life – start living it
… Life is carrying you, holding your hand, knowing what
you need … high time to celebrate … all is included …

Chapter 6

Your creativity and potential are the invisible divine!

To allow your to Your inner potential and creativity to
unfold and flower. Expanding in awareness, Witnessing
your inner true abundance to unfold …

Chapter 7

Relaxing into silence … it knows!

Presence, the invisible, the unknown, the silence that is
behind and in it all … Just allow that wisdom to embrace
you. ! Blissful living, is being you and flowing with what
is…to embrace and be embraced by the whole.

Chapter 1

The invitation, stop running away from yourself!

**The invitation, our greatest adventure begins
within … stop running away.
You are the friend you been waiting for.
Just stop and enter into the here and now … to be
present and aware is to start living an authentic life.
To move from person to presence. To understand
you are born to be you, no one else.**

The first and only important step to take is to stop into presence. In this now the whole eternity is hiding. There is nowhere to go. Even if we think so in our running. It is like we are running away from our self into something we don't know what is it. This is a misunderstanding. We have forgot the source we all are. That is within us. Now is the time to come home and turn within. Connect, finding where all you ever want, has its answers, like a forgotten treasure box. As within so without. So if you long for different outcome in your life, successes in your work, happier self, and a more loving relationship, all that will have its start by you meeting you within. There it all has its beginning. Also the spiritual self… is to be found there. Living life as an awakening process…

To move from personality into presence. You are the only one who can fulfill your dreams, and visions to come true and be free and alive. No one else can do this.

It is all in your hands. This book is about awakening into that possibility.

Bliss is 'living in endless abundance'
True wealth starts here and now within your own source...

'Life is available only in the present moment ...' Osho

Stop running away, you are the friend you have been waiting for. The way to true success is to meet your own inner self, the greatest adventure you will ever meet.

Be the leader of your own life. Since bliss, true abundance and transformation can only happen in presence, your greatest adventure begins here and now. To step into presence and to stay there, is of great importance of transformation and inner leadership. We have never been, and will never be anywhere else than here. This presence is all there is and ever will be. We just need to stop and built a friendship to it. But we all run away from our self. Do you have any idea what you are running away from? I had no idea once. I did know better. I had no clue that presence and turning within could help me in my life. Now I know for sure that it is the only way.

To realize that and to start breathing and to start listen, is the first gift to lead of your self.. To start being true to yourself, to sort your self up, finding true abundance and success. It doesn't matter how fast you run if you are running in the wrong direction. Better stop and tune within for the right direction first.

This is to reach your own truth, highest potential and to understand that the magic source of it all is within you. Stop and connect within, meeting your own source and magic self. As within so without. Here you start to create and relax in your own life.

What are we fighting in life, and why? Pain, love, money issues, fear, low self-confidence ... feelings, longings ... we all have a little of everything. We closed the door to all that we carry within into turning the energy without ourself hoping to get what we long for from the outer world.

And all of this can only be healed by stopping to run away and to turn within yourself, by bringing awareness and love. That is what this whole book is about .

We are like a rock that has been skipping on the surface of the ocean, not being able to stop. When it stops and drops into the ocean, it starts moving into the magic of it all. Without any problems, it sinks by itself. The same is true of us. Our mind has become like the surface of the ocean. It thinks, it knows, it analyses, it thinks in terms of right and wrong … it tries to control and it takes all magic away. The opposite is so magical, blissful, abundant, joyous and peaceful.

The mind always lives in the past or focuses on the future with all our dreams and worries. To stop and to drop is to turn from the mind Into your heart, feeling your self and truth..

Turn around and find that all you experience in life is within. As within, so without, it all starts here, nowhere else. To connect within is to start meeting all. To be in this presence is all there is … When meeting yourself and your life, start transforming. In running away, you only suffer and miss the point.

My life experience dropping into now

I asked for help, it came and new life started to guide me …

In one specific moment in my life, it all changed. Not that I had any idea of that then … I moved from living from my mind into living from my heart. It just cracked open one working almost 40 years ago.

It started with me falling onto the bedroom floor one early morning being alone at home before going to work. I just by it self, fell down crying in despair, asking for help, something I never had done before. Without knowing or expecting anything, my life was in that moment starting to change. I had cracked open from within, a longing heart that had just opened into nothing as it looked. I dried my tears after a really "giving it all" Feeling, and went to work as if nothing had happened.

Without being aware or knowing I had surrendered to something bigger than myself.

My stopping and dropping was and still is a blessing in my life.

My pain after a missing mother and her death a few years earlier was making me run – faster and faster…

Since her death, when I was 20, and even before that I had I been hiding all pain I was carrying within me. It had been a life journey with pretending that my feelings was not important at all, others where. I did hide mine. I did not even know I had them… It was making me run faster and faster away from myself. I fell in love, got married, and got divorced after a few years. I was not there at all. I had a panic attack when my husband started to talk about children… me children… me who never even liked to play with dolls… I was just surviving… all became chaotic within.

Now at 27, I was living with a new man. . I had collected so much pain I was so unaware, just pushing me to run and not having any needs. Just push my inner self down. At this point, nothing in the so-called outer world mattered to me any longer. A void of emptiness and pain was within me, and an aching heart was hunting me with nightmares filled with guilt. Me just trying to avoid the situation until it all stopped.
I don't think we are so different… we all carry pain that we hide.
This morning in my life was like My heart was just cracking within me, like a seed that is letting go of its shell … This happening with all its crying was, without me being aware of it, a new start in my life. I asked crying in despair for help and it started to come….

The moment we open the door to this innocence, the love and intelligence of the soul is there … and it knows.

Intellectual knowledge can be of great help, but it will not transform your life and not open you to the magic and mysteries of existence.

My asking in a total surrender to something bigger was without any thought or knowing.. it was pure happening and a blessing.

I was not aware of how much I had taken on my shoulders … From childhood and beyond … an inner feeling that everything was my fault.

When I stopped on the floor crying, presence stepped in, I later started to realize that problem never existed in the now … I had cracked open like a seed and a new life was opened up for me. A crying for help, I asked for, just a call for help … to something bigger than me, something unknown … in this surrender, trust was born. Trust of something invisible … I had given up…

Starting to get an understanding about what I needed to do, guided by the here and now, coming to me I started to feel trust and the absence of a path … a calmness within.

From this morning on, I could see that life started to guide me in a new direction … it had all stopped and I knew deep inside that there was more to life than this. I knew it because I had an old feeling from early in life when I lived in trust.

So to stop and drop beyond the mind into the presence. To surrender to something bigger was the first step for me, to receive help that silently started to come was the second, from this point steps were being taken without me being in control of them.

At first, nothing in the outer world changed … it was just all within me. To begin with just feeling me.

Today I call this presence being authentic … living, trusting and taking one step at a time. To be able to respond, following the heart and my own perfect inner knowing and agenda, not following others. In union with others as it came to be.

Today I enjoy presence and bliss in the ordinary things in life, drinking a glass of water, taking a shower … just pure bliss moments … allowing my feet to walk me, I follow … to feel my body … all this a call to trust what is … Within as without … confident being a leader in my own life, to celebrate it.

I am not unique in this way. We all have a longing inside to wake up and to be who we are here to be. We need to start feeling us, start to listen to ourselves deeper … starting to stand on our own side … stop being a pleaser to others.

In all group processes, retreats, coaching sessions and leadership trainings I conduct, even if there is structure around it, every step is in the now moment, a natural expansion is then naturally happening, into who we truly are … moment by moment. So it is high time to let go of holding yourself back. To start opening up and to feel. Never be afraid of a breakdown … of crying, it can be turned into a breakthrough and a turning point in your life.

In that way, a new life and transformation can happen. From here to the next here. Deepening within.

Connecting within is to move from the mind into our energy, into feeling us, reaching our heart and being. It is a journey with a beginning but with no end … me falling onto the floor was a starting point … all stopped … my mind was giving up its controlling system. I just did not want to continue on that path any longer, and I guess you feel the same or have had the same experience.

A step often happens when something is pushing us. It can be as it was for me. It can be carrying so much pain inside that you can't handle it. Or a dear loved one gets sick, a child is hurt or someone dies.

A step can happen in many different ways – a divorce, you get hurt in different aspects of your life, you lose your job – drastic or slowly. We all have met it in different ways. Sometimes we can handle it, and when it is too much, we may have a panic attack or our heart starts to beat fast. Life as such is insecure, so to trying control life, yourself and others is hopeless.

The teaching is to find out who you are not, so you can start finding out who you are. And it all starts here and now. You don't need to know, or cannot know how; you can just start trusting. Never fight what has pushed you. Instead, just thank it. It will bring you into transformation.

That life is here for you now … and what is now is the starting point, the diving in point … nowhere else … believing that the grass is greener somewhere else is to escape, to avoid. As with all addictions, they are just a substitute for meeting you. It is maybe the best for you so far … but when turning within yourself, starting to embrace you, understanding what you have been closing off in there, you will start changing, not by doing but by feeling more and more your own truth.

You are the friend you have been waiting for. To start meeting, feeling and unravelling yourself as a starting point but no end … it is an endless journey.

We have been trusting the outer world, been running other people's agendas and needs … now it is more important than ever to know your own needs and longings since the world is showing us its fragile side.

The best part in all this is that all we ever long for is already here within … nowhere else … we have forgotten, and the focus has been lost in the outer world. Now is the time to rise in awareness and consciousness.

To meet yourself. To start meeting all-loving good energy you truly are.. Beyond all stressful thoughts. To understand this is to start transforming your life. The key is to move from thinking you into the feeling and being you… To open your loving eyes into the present moment, is the key forever. It is all waiting for you here, to discover the depth we usually run away from. To move from thinking us and life. Beyond the past and the future. To start to use life as an awakening process.

If you, for a moment, just stop here and now … maybe sit down, become aware of your body and your breathing. Have a gap in your reading …

Feel your feet … Feel your breathing opening and expanding within you …

Just notice what is going on in this very moment … allow an expansion to happen …

Just knowing that your body, your breathing is always here and now … feeling you is always here and now … to move from personality into presence, being without any idea … just feeling you … allowing you … all you ever experienced in life is there., all memories. Don't push just know for now.

Maybe there is a longing deep within … nothing you need to do … just feel it, and trust it. It is like the inner part of a flower seed.

When the shell cracks, it will start growing by itself … you cannot do this. You can only allow it.

Step by step we going deeper into understanding, like the rock falling deeper into the magic of the ocean, accepting, expanding into awareness … allowing the true self to come to the surface … always in the here-and-now moment. This is how I run my groups, retreats and sessions.

Life is available only in the present moment. Be grateful for all that comes to you; embrace, feel and accept everything this moment brings to you for growth. Trust your inner longing. It knows something. So connect within yourself.

To ask for help is a sign of strength when being vulnerable, in pain and in a feeling of being lost. I call this presence the true possibility to live and create your blissful reality, melting into what is.

In my life experience

To stop running away from my self, was the magic moment. To ask for help is a key, and the here and now listens. In this, a life long transformation started.

Living in the now I call living in the wisdom of the soul.Authentic living.

To stop living from the mind and having stressful thoughts and to drop into your heart is the first step of transformation … This is to start an authentic life. So easy and so rewarding. Just remember, stop asking for answers and confirmation without; instead, start listening to your inner. It knows.

The heart is silently and patiently waiting for you.

Meditation or Awareness Practice

Just stop … breath and feel this moment… …close your eyes and move within … all you seek and all answers will come at the perfect time.

If you were to ask for help, what would it be for?

'Tomorrow will never happen, it never comes, it is always today'. — Osho

Chapter 2

The bigger picture, the big magic!

**Lift your eyes, look at the sky, see the empty space
beyond all the clouds … it has a message for you.**

We are pure universal consciousness in a human body form, so much more than we ever think or ever believe. In this connection all becomes possible. To understand we are meant to be here. You are invited by the whole. To experience this whole through being a human being is our gift to ourselves. In this, we have a possibility to expand and to live fully. In this vast pure connection, all becomes possible. To connect with the source, to open the channel of energy flow within us, always connected, no sprain exist.

Like a fountain, we are all connected to the whole universe, endlessly abundant! When we understand and trust that we can look much more easy at our self, feeling our self with more clear eyes….without putting any ideology on to it.. just letting it be open in the here and know…

Bliss is living in this connection, being a
channel with endless true possibilities.

Bliss is 'living in endless abundance'.
True wealth starts within, connecting to the universal source itself …

'The universe reveals its secrets to those who dare to follow their hearts'.

To understand that we all are pure universal consciousness, belonging to this universe. To open your eyes and see the endless sky with all its stars. You, yourself, are a reflection of the stars you see.

Become aware of the synchronicity…

The second step of understanding is to open up to the big something. We often think we are alone here, separated from the whole. We are not. We are invited here. But we have forgot. So to remember breathing can be of big help, then we connect. To open up yourself to something bigger … to become a blissful leader in your own life. I once had the idea that I was alone and separated. That was to live in constant pain, believing I was not wanted here. Now I know by experiences, that the opposite is true, we are all invited to this all inclusive life journey.

When we live in separation from the bigger something, we make ourselves small. Lose our confidence. In opening up to the bigger picture of this endless universe, our separation goes away and endless possibilities come into our life. To open yourself to the whole universe, you start building trust, and everything becomes possible. Just here and now to take it in.

To understand we are aligned with the whole. To feel we belong to a bigger truth than just our own little world. This will make the fear go away, the fear of being alone and separated.

For me, this was the first step to build trust. To see that I belong here. That made me, even if unaware then, start to see myself as a part of a bigger something. The energy we are came from and always is in connection.

To see the bigger picture makes it possible to see yourself in a brighter light – a light we truly are. You are bigger than the body … as big as the whole universe. We are the consciousness within it all.

'The body does not contain you; in fact, you contain the body. Ordinarily you think, "I exist in the body". This is absolutely wrong. The body exists in you; you are vaster, you are bigger – not only bigger than the body, but also you are bigger than this whole universe. It is awareness that holds all'. – Osho

Everything in this universe is moving in synchronicity, in perfect order.

We just don't see that. Becoming aware, we start trusting something we can't understand, we can only witness. Someone once told me that life is like an empty canvas to be painted on … you are the brush and the universe is the consciousness that is holding it. We think we are the doer of it all … yet we are not … we are the co-worker to the whole … we are just a traveller witnessing it all. In the endless possibilities that are there or here. Trust and expand in this presence.

Since we are universal energy, it attracts and repels. So to live in alignment within, you can attract more and more through your heart's longing.

In my life experience...

I remembered and started to understand to space out, and to space in. We are all aligned with the whole...

After falling down on the floor, I started to become aware of the response, and new events that perfectly started to come into my life. My nightmares guided me to seek answers and synchronistic events started to become visible for me. ... and it made me seek deeper meaning in life ... past life, why all this guilt? Looking at the midnight sky made me wonder ...

My inner self was in turmoil, no doubt about that ... my nightmares were killing me ... at the same time, I could see help was coming to me. I did not know where to look for it and to become aware, that it happened to me ... was magic ... books about initiation, earlier life, that we are not our body, it is our temple for a while, all kinds of new information. It was like something in me started to open up to new, or old, ideas and possibilities.

I started to question ... my dreams ... my mother was always in the dreams, my guilt ... what was it all about ...? Just me questioning was a help ... the dream was slowly changing into 'nicer' aspects on the same theme ...What was it my inner self wanted to tell? I was starting to question and watching my self from without and a higher place...

I started to use my alone time as a 'kind of meditation', even if I did not have any ideas about it then.

I was just on my sofa ... alone at home ... spacing out ... or was I spacing in ... I don't know , it was a beginning of expanding and to meditate. – it was all in one. This gave me insights. I don't know how long I was in this space but it was for hours ...

I started to see my childhood ... and I started to understand the guilt feelings ... they did not disappear but I could understand ...

I remember me before all inner doors were closing, a very trusting innocent little girl. Happy being in nature ... trusting and in silent communion.

One clear strong memory came to me one day. I remembered me sitting by a fountain waiting for my mother who was shopping. I was about four or five years old. The sun was glittering on the water of a fountain. Me looking, being present, seeing the beauty endlessly reflecting. I just remembered that at that moment, I understood that we all are like fountains, just pouring out endless energy. At that moment, I saw people passing by with sad faces. Why were they not happy? I asked my mother about this when she came back, but she could not give me any answers. This question had been there all these years and now this fountain of light was starting to come alive.

As a child Up until five I was open.. then I also started to close since life around me, in my family was to painful for me. Sitting by the fountain open and innocent I could see that everyone had forgotten about the divine light within and the endless possibility that exists.

Now I had become one of them. Now to start opening myself up and to start remember was a release.

So much had happened since then, where I had closed all inner doors. Now to open up again.. starting to understand. It all was interconnected. I had closed and now it was starting to open up.

Understanding … that existence wants me here … that's the truth. No one of us can argue about that. Gave me a space to look at my own story.

Beyond my own understanding. It was all so perfect and always came in such perfect order that my mind could not go into fighting it.

A silent presence was more and more embracing me. Nothing dramatic happened … I was still going to work … living with my partner, but my inner life was coming more and more alive. New people, meetings … people and books, relaxing music and so on were perfectly fitting into my life. I was not a seeker, but something was starting to guide me. I felt it like a fountain that had been closed for the winter and that was now opening up. And the more we trust it and open up to it, the more the impossible becomes the possible.

We all contain light and darkness. It works within us. We are all energy, not only parts.

Bring light into the dark and it disappears … being into the love and it expands. In awareness. this is in our hands.

I could start seeing that existence was bringing me new energy after me falling to the floor that morning. Learning to become one with my breathing … to understand that breathing is the bridge and the door between the inner and outer universe. To keep the connection alive with all its endless possibilities …

I read books about different initiations, past lives … and I started to meditate within the bigger something, just by myself. I had dates every Saturday morning with existence. That gave me comfort, and memories started to come to the surface.

Consciousness is all there is … knowing your being is endless.

For me, when creating transforming group processes, it is important to built trust.. to open up to the bigger something. Otherwise, we are identified with the 'painful experiences' of me, myself and I, as a separated unity. Since we are not, it is important to see ourselves from a higher point of view.

Rising in awareness. Becoming aware of the big magical mysteries… the energy behind and within all form. To know that Our heart and this universe are responding to each other. For me, this is what I have been walking on. To be alive and open. Always into the highest order. To trust me to be me, you to be you. To manifest dreams. This is so we can see the invisible behind it all … the dance with the universe is like that.As I see it.

Energy moves between polarities. And we contain it all..so there is no good and bad, right and wrong.. it is just polarities. So when we open up we open to it all. We better learn to live it all, not to be identified with a part.

Your inner longing and the will of the universe, move hand in hand … so trust this and do not allow thoughts to stand in the way. For me, this has been the most important thing to be aware of … and as a child, it was so natural … we all have this innocence and deep trust within somewhere …

We all come and are this universal consciousness. We are all born out of this magic … with no beginning and no end … our mind can't understand it, but our heart's wisdom knows. There we can open and feel it. Like an innocent child feels the miracle of it all. Start trusting your endless loving heart.

Open the channel to the whole universe … then you can create and live aligned in true success … and truth itself. Moving from fear and separation into trusting and being in connection happen when we stop, bring rareness and low us to receive.

We all come from the same source. When we were born, we had the connection naturally within us … then slowly, slowly we started to identify with the outer world. Now is the time to start remembering again …

You belong to the universe. Universal consciousness, experiencing being in a human body. Beyond all or beliefs. To come back to this innocence again … to open up and trust so our life can expand in a way we long for.
We are all pure energy, divine light. In letting go of our old concepts, love starts to flow …
This divine light, when it starts to be free of old ideas and pains, free from disharmony … begins coming alive … we feel love, feel

acceptance, we can be alive and live our self in a true way. It is all happening in perfect synchronicity.

I started to become aware of that. With new awareness and openness I could understand my dreams and they changed… The guilt was letting go, but the source of the problem remains within me… but my willingness to clear my own inner was I hint that lessened the unconscious mind to be so dramatic. I could start to follow my inner guiding.

I am no good in dreams. I just know my dreams went from being horrible to be more guiding in a positive way.

I had open the door to my inner… I had open my eyes to the bigger something .. trust was expanding. The magic of life it self had started to happen.

For me, this was important to understand before the next step was going to take place. And I think for all of us, when looking into ourselves, to find the bigger connection is important. Not to be identified with parts, especially painful parts. We are consciousness … this consciousness is connected with the whole universe … in this we can become free. and the one we are meant to be. A truer you and me.

Always trust the inner energy … it knows … follow it and you will follow truth.

The energy knows what the mind does not.

Even if we have closed the door and started to mistrust … know that the door is there … we can open it again … when time is right and ripe. Built trust…

When we live with the idea that we are lacking certain qualities, we feel a need. It is our mind that tries to take our attention instead of living from our trusting heart.

Synchronicity … we are all in this together …

Breathing is the bridge and a natural part of opening up to the bigger, a bridge between your inner and outer sky.

This way your trust grows.

I know, because this became my truth … stepping out of my own way … I became aware as synchronistic events started to happen … In this way, life shifts dimensions …

Trusting your inner self, it knows it has just been closed for a while. We all come from the same source … before body … no body … after body … no body … essence or consciousness itself … for now a human experience in a body. . That's the gift and the invitation. Meditation helps this To become true and visible.

In Short My Experience

To be in connection within, is to be open to the divine .Re-connect and start to re- member … In this I know we have the possibility to heal ourself. To become whole again.

Today I call this living in trust, in connection, open and aware, trusting the endless possibilities and longing contained within. We are given the experience of being a consciousness in a human form.

I call this today living in alignment, vertical. In this bliss, true abundance has its roots.

Meditation and Awareness Practice

Look at the sky and focus on the endless space between the clouds … Become aware about how life present it self in perfect order, called synchronicity.

'We are the whole ocean in a dew drop, not the dew drop in the ocean …' — Rumi

Chapter 3

Emotional healing, clearing the past!

Stepping out of your own way. To live in the here
and now without being blinded by the past.
To clear the inner space from the old holding you back …
To become aware of what you are carrying within.
What is holding you back from living.
Nothing was ever your fault and you are not a
victim here, even if you think and feel so …
Bring light and awareness into your story. Transformation
is then starting to happen. From feeling pain,
you will find your truth, love and freedom.

To free yourself, stepping beyond the mind and the old …
master your life with a healthy mind and open
heart … finding your truth … Transform the past
into free energy, wisdom and harmony.
'Bliss living' is to clear what is standing in your way …
Imagine a garage or storage so filled with
stuff that you can't use it anymore …

Bliss 'living in endless abundance'
True wealth starts with stepping out of your own way …

'The only problem with sadness, desperateness, anger, hopelessness, anxiety, misery, is that you want to get rid of them. That's the only barrier. You will have to live them. They are the very situation in which life has to integrate and grow'. – Osho The Art of Dying, Talk #10

Step out of your own way, making space for you to live you, in freedom, and the loving potential and harmony you truly are.

The third very important step, as it was for me is to step out of your own way. To realize that the truth of you is not in the pain of the old story, that we have identified our self with. We are all living in a survival mood, not being free from old wounds that we carry within. To become aware of your inner self, beyond the story we need to see and feel what we carrying from the past. To clear it, is to look into it. To feel it not thinking it. Wanting to free our self, to feel good and live an abundant true, prosperous life – the third part of inner leadership – we need to bring our inner child back home again, into its wisdom and pure power.

I once did not have a clue that turning within was possible, and that it would not only heal me, but also give me freedom and a blissful life. That it would transform me. To bring light within, meeting and embrace the feelings we are carrying. To stop living in separation.. To move from the mind and its painful separating thoughts and it's painful feelings into truth and the healing heart. Clearing the inner self is to embrace and bring awareness into it.

We can not become free by just thinking it.. we need to feel it fully so it can be healed.energy move in circles and when it has stoped mid ways … we need to feel it fully.

This is needed so we do not hold ourselves back in a separation mood any longer. Thoughts, old feelings, guilt, resentment, all this pain is freedom and love up side down. To put is right again so life energy can flow. We are all carrying a story. We are born into different family situation. It is like we are born onto a stage where a play or a drama has been going on long before we entered. It is not how it all started that matters … it is how we can handle our life now that matters. Like cleaning a garage or storage unit that so it can been used for its own purpose again.

We are, when born, just divine energy in a body, let's come back to that trusting wisdom. There and then we needed attention and help from the outside. Now it is a new situation.

No matter how it looked, it has formed us. Usually, it is said that by the time we are five, we have created a survival strategy. It is not something we knew about then, but we can start seeing it now. Up until five, we are just energy and feelings, and then around four or five we have created a system that we use to 'survive'.unconsciously. Now time to become conscious again.

We have needed a strategy to avoid our pain, we all do that until we understand that there is healing path that will lead us into our true self. I use to say, that all children are super intelligent in intuition and always create the best ways for survival. Now we can wake up beyond that old strategy. That was then, To carry these patterns is to hold your energy stuck in an old form. To start to release yourself, to step out of your old mindset, To start feeling you.. to bring the feelings into the loving ness within you. To free yourself. To give yourself a second birth, I am simply saying that there is a way to be sane … That you can start seeing and handling what has been created by the past in you. Start witnessing your inner thought process and what that makes you feel.

As human beings we all have a mind with thoughts that come and go and repeat themselves … you can be aware of them or not. To become aware is to wake up and to have choices.
All thoughts are connected to beliefs. To bring awareness is an important step towards transformation and free living.

In my life experience...

I needed to bring light into all the pain … and the old story.

I was guided to take my own pain into my own hands, the greatest of gift. I was unaware of the inner, unhealthy mind and energy system. So much pain. Not to fear my inner feelings and pain, anymore. No more hiding behind guilt and sorrow. It was not about the past or the other, it was only about finding me, and to be whole, to come home.

I was guided and recommended to a transforming therapeutical awakening process by a doctor I visited him for various problems. He just told me that I needed help. I had no idea what he was talking about but I felt he was right. He told me to work on my inner self. To connect again other wise I would be more sick an die like my mother. She had a brain tumor and he asked me if she was carrying a lot of sadness. My answers was a clear yes.. That sadness killed her, he said. You better take care of that sadness within you other wise you also continue to close all these feelings within you. I knew he was right. It was like my whole system knew something I did not.

A registered for the program the doctor recommended.
From my parents divorce where no one said anything, or talked about it, my mother leaving the family. I was ten. I was the youngest in the family. My brothers were 11 and 13 when I was born. They were more aware of what had happened … but not me. I was born when my mother was on her way to starting to work after years of being a housewife and taking care of two sons. I was unconsciously blamed for it all. Something I never thought about before I started a transforming process. To understand and look into what had happened. To see it from all corners and understand me and the others.
To start questioning and to bring light into all inner corners. It was not about them, it was about me.. what I felt, what I had experienced, where I had closed off…. just to see that the burden of that was holding me in the grip of running so fast to compensate. The morning I fell on the floor, I did not know anything about this, but something deep inside me had a strong longing to break free and

to start remembering who I was before all the closing down started. For 12 weeks I was in this 'self towards awareness rebirth' (STAR) process. A real waker-upper.

We were supposed to write our story down, all the years starting from birth, to understand and look from without on it … we were breathing to feel, and we were feeling I cried endlessly like a cleansing. I think I after this process cried for three years … so much was suppressed. We were guided lovingly and with awareness, and we started to meditate. I really fell in love with that. The meditations we did really helped me build a space within me where I could rest. Like the outer blissful space I knew about also was within me.

I was pushed, guided and I jumped and took all the leaps possible to look into the dark corners of my inner self. To be in a process like this is just to be guided and to follow. It all happens by itself. I had never been even thinking about therapy, not being a seeker or longing for some kind of spiritual work. But did I feel good, healed and thankful for the process. I loved every part of it. In the beginning, it was difficult to put words to it … but in the process, it was so easy and so tremendously helpful. I started to relate to my own story. I was afraid of it. Especially when I could see I was repeating the patterns. When I was asked if I wanted to have children when I was young, I had a panic attack. It was like something within me knew that I did not want to repeat the pattern of being an unwanted child.

This process of meeting me, embracing me, forgiving me, crying me, feeling me, understanding me, took me out of 'the bottle' (my mind and all its thoughts..) … it was never any ones faults.. my mothers or fathers, brothers or relatives, they where them self hurt and unaware. I just felt light, free and could start breathing.

All of this experiences and more I include in my transforming group process today. … we can't know ourselves and others if we don't look under the surface. Here is the place where transformation happen. And it is so natural. As diving Under the surface of the ocean.

Never fear your feelings … move into them, allow them, and it will be transformed. Always accept with loving aware support.

My inquiring stepping out of my way was to step in … bringing light, awareness, looking into all the pains and corners … starting to feel me …looking at old believes. Feeling the truth or not in them now.

In the beginning of life, we are only energy and feeling. No mind … when we became a bit older the mind comes in … first feeling, then thought … now we need to go back to feel again and find the truth. This is transformation … to feel, to heal and to start finding truth now. To feel and heal us to open your heart again. Once it was open as children, and we slowly closed it to survive: Now it is time to open it again. For yourself finding freedom.

I am so grateful and happy for being guided and pushed in the direction of meeting myself. This is why I share my story today.

To embrace your inner, to stop fighting it … to bring awareness and light with a lot of help from transforming meditation techniques that I was guided to.

All dramas contain three different qualities… Just look at any movie you see in life… this is called the Karpman triangle.

There is a victim, and a strong controlling person that controls the drama and some one that wants to sort it out, a helper.

In a family, or company in society these qualities are played out..

When we start to heal and forgive all this energies will meet within your self. Like you start to feel your own power and direction, you allow yourself to be vulnerable and since you are reading this book you a are stepping into helping yourself and be on your own side… When you become more and more aware of this you will find it very inspiring. In what triangle do I step in.. or what triangle am I playing out. Just become aware.

Where we are in the world today … as I see it, more or less need to make this shift … to understand and know who we are. To stop bringing pain onto ourself and on to others. To come home and to bring true love and awareness to ourselves again. As human beings, we have the possibility of opening our hearts, opening to the wisdom and alive healing we all contain within. To be responsible, to sort ourselves out.
To stop blaming others for your pain, that is only bringing war into your life and not any peace or healing.

Being a leader, taking your own life into your hands … not fearing the feelings of the old … they are the soil to grow in, into being your true self.

Your feelings to be embraced will only create empathy for others – a very healthy quality when working and living with people.

To clear your own path is the first step towards your own successes in life. To be responsible.

Nothing is personal in this life drama … only to clear the energy and life will respond in a new way.

By seeing, you start transforming. Accept help from aware people who can hold your hand. That is what I see my job Is al about …
All you can do is to bring light into the dark corner of your being. This is how to sort out what is true now, and what is standing in your way. To be free in finding your own truth to live, to live in this that I call bliss …

We all have the possibility to start shining our inner light. We all can do this. You can't shine somebody else's light. Awareness is putting light onto yourself here and now … no judging … just a curiosity to meet and experience yourself. Accept help … be supported and trust that you are already the one you are here to be … it is all hiding within you.

Whatever pain and miserable story you are carrying it is actually over, and the longing in your heart is a mystery to be lived so it all can be healed.

For now, relax and practice trust. We have lost our way and …now we can start finding it again.

Forgiveness is without morality. It is to let go of what is no longer is serving you. I always include a forgiveness and letting go ceremony in my retreats … this is one of the important steps to take, a willingness to let go of old identifications. From holding on to being right to being free and happy. You choose. A willingness to heal, letting go is a solution for your freedom.

In Short My Experience

It is necessary to face, bring light and embrace all your inner painful experiences. That will be like bringing light into the whole energy system In this I started to free my self from old concepts and believes. Not only my body became healthy, my mind and my heart too. To step into my true self was loving medicine for my whole being.
In this my self-confidence and truth grows.

Meditation and Awareness Practice

Who would you be without your story? The pain is in the identification with thoughts and feelings that is not looked into yet. Mind, open heart and being …

Write your story down so you can start to understand. Forgive the people in it when you can… they where all most probably unaware …

'Without your story you are perfectly sane …'– Byron Katie

Chapter 4

The radiance of love you truly are!

Trusting your own heart … Loving yourself, your partner and others. To value presence in endless bliss and abundance …

Living love is to live in true abundance. Love lives in every cell of
our body … we are love…the only thing fighting it, is our mind.
Live the goodness you truly are … it is always in the present
moment, nowhere else, and it is to be shared and trusted.
Love is a quality, not a relationship. This quality is medicine and
healing for your whole system. The radiance in you is pure love,
healing all aspects of your life! Share it, live it … abundantly so …
wealth, health and abundance can happen … It all goes together.
Open your heart … it is pure love in different forms
… from attraction to compassion to devotion.
Love is the strongest power In the world…

Bliss 'living in endless abundance'
True wealth starts within your own heart and its source …

Your task is not to seek for love, but merely to seek and find all barriers that you have built against it.' — Rumi

You are, we all are love … love is our true nature … we don't 'need' love, we are love. Feel it and share it. In this way, we can start living in harmony with what is! Your heart is endlessly abundant, and all wealth goes together with it. Inner union and outer union goes together …

To listen to your heart's wisdom and its truth is a very important part in inner leadership. In that we can respect others. We all have this possibility to do so. To realize we are pure divine energy, an energy that is innocence, accepting, present and goodness. To start listening to your heart, is wisdom.. Bring your thoughts to your heart. There truth and new wisdom will be found. We usually take our love to the mind and start analyzing it. Then we lose it, and the magic is gone .. Today I see love as the solution for most things… together with meditation it is pure healing medicine.

To start looking within to find it. We all are it… we just need to look. Just right now take a few moments to meditate on what love is for you. Feel it… if it is for some one, it doesn't matter it is felt within you.

We have all lived strange life's the last year. Separated from each other. In one way that has a gift. The gift is that we have to look deeper within our self to find a deeper connection. In our heart where we find love for our self and others we never need to feel separated. So in this sense we have all been trained to drop within our self for solutions. Finding deeper truth and direction.

As a child you were only innocent, and love was natural and alive.. To come back to that again, to remember. Inner leadership is to be in connection with the energy of the heart and to bring awareness into what is. In pure acceptance, exploring its wisdom. That is pure power. In this, you will start melting within as without. To live from our open heart is to live in true abundance. Your heart's wisdom and the voice of truth guide us. Love is always happening in the present moment, so always accepting what is, without judgement.

We have in our life stopped trusting love and instead started to control and put ideas onto ourselves, our life and onto others. Love has become an idea, not a reality to live. We often say you can't trust love, and this is so true … it is alive and it has its own way. But often we have not stopped and inquired what love is. It is an energy within presence, not a concept.

Living with an open heart, understanding yourself, you will experience the love you truly are. The energy that is within us is goodness. A love that is abundant and filled with its own wisdom. To start experiencing that you are love and do not need love from outside is such a big gift. You are a whole human being, not the parts of one. The first step in this is to love ourselves.

To live in alignment with love is to open your heart, resting in it, to feel the truth and wisdom there. Our heart is the transformer within us.

Since love is energy and moves between polarities , it attracts and it repels. So through loving yourself and Including all parts, you are moving into more and harmony, and in this you attract more love. . Find your shining star within your heart, and share it. ...

Love without awareness becomes one sided... awareness without love becomes one sided. So bring awareness into love... and bring love into your awareness. Otherwise we easy bring conditions and ideas to loved. In that way we lose connection with it. We close the door to . Love is natural and it is always present, here and now. Let it be alive and moving. It knows what you mind has lost. So the first step is to love yourself. Nothing else is possible. To live love liberates you ...

To see what love is when you are at work. Do you feel passion for what you do? Do you feel great full for the people you work with? Are able to be honest .. Do loving your self bring your true capacity into what you do?

What is love in your relationships... How many different types of love is there... Love can be in all aspects of your life... How do you tell people that you participate them.. We are miserly telling positive feelings.. And to your self.. do you give yourself credit and love for what you do...? Start to do that ... for being brave .. for being honest... for daring ..etc...

In my life experience …

Love is the silent force that is running behind all the noise within me. Your heart is the door…

Form, is the biggest act of love towards your self . Open up, to trust the bigger something and to clear the old from a free flowing energy. If we don't free us within, we stop the flow, we get sick and stop ourself from living love.

For me love is not a reflation ship. It is who I am, and in that, relating is included. Different aspects in different areas. Attraction and sex between couples. Loving the I am in the business world.

Emotional freedom is love for me… to live my own truth is love. To trust in my self and to feel confidence within. Devotion when it came to surrendering. All different aspects from attraction into compassion and devotion.

After the big cleansing transforming group process I went through. A stronger presence was there… and love. The energy started to go low and to guide me. Before my therapeutical rains formation I was often sick. Not in "big" important ways, but it could lead to it. Now I could feel the aliveness within me.. very rarely sick, love life and free flowing energy is the medicine. Happy me, happy body, happy you.

I was starting to expand. This true energy of love was and is filling me from within. Like layers of the old was falling of me. Big changes just happened. Trust was there and love towards what wanted to come. My open heart was starting to guide me. It was guiding me in new ways, into more and more compassion, and later into devotion …

To bring awareness into my life was of biggest importance. Love and meditation goes together.

I started to love and respect me. I had gone from thinking me to feeling and being me. It all just happened so naturally and easy. Like my inner was guiding me into higher levels of my self.

I started to see and follow love as the natural force within us all.. I started to respect my self… It has taken me many many years to be able to words on to this. It has just been a trusting Inner feeling.

When love is blocked and controlled by the mind, it is painful, and sickening. The door to the heart is closed. Then we think we need it from without. When we live open it is flowing from within. No more need. To trust the inner heart. Is to respect and love my self. In this a magical life starts.

I had always been 'falling' in love. It all started already when I was five. Since then relating had been followed. When identified with the past they ended in pain. When more and more moving in awareness and love, it is still pain there, but a loving friendliness always follows.

More and more a rising in love instead of the falling.
Now I felt compassion for myself and others too.

I fell in love with meditation, the once we had done in the transforming process … this meditation led me to a centre in Stockholm that was facilitating the meditation. I found myself going there.

One day, I was listening to the master who had created and updated meditation for the modern man. Just by listening, my heart melted. I cannot say what happened … only a feeling of 'finally' someone is sharing the truth … In this moment I kind of knew that my heart had a connection, and knew something that was beyond my earlier experiences. A devotion beyond it all. An new kind of invisible love affair started. I had experienced different love affairs where my heart had opened. But never like this … it was a whole different experience and sensation.

In relationships, one's partner always wants something … here it was clean and clear. It was all within me.

This devotion made me experience something I never thought possible. To come back home in bliss. Living in grace with what is. It was never without me … it just needed to be remembered and mirrored.

Listening to truth speaking and feeling the light within. Meeting this master, was magical, meeting grace, light, a light that was within me.. Since my life journey changed into more ways of awareness in life, my so-called love life also changed. It became more fulfilling. The most important part of my life was expanding. I went to the United States and later to India and met Osho in person.

To melt into his presence is beyond words for me. It melted everything in my life, and is still doing so. Melting into awareness, becoming an Osho therapeutical counsellor, a meditation facilitator.

Sitting at his feet in silence, and celebrating what was happening for some years. It was a blessing beyond all words. I carry and live that, now long after Osho left his body. There is no difference in the inner connection. I can't put into words Onto this divine experience other than to say, it is an endless love affair within me, silently and divine presents. Silence, love, aliveness, awareness, dancing in this endless bliss. Devotion is a higher form of love … in this all other love affairs happen.

The wisdom of the heart is always present, and it was waiting for me to take my next step – into living and sharing this devotion. This wisdom of the heart always knows. It has a connection with a deeper source than we understand and know.

I never thought that this would be my life in the outside world … Even if I took as many long trainings as possible and was asked to assist in groups, it was never in my mind to work as a group leader or counseling therapist.

A silent happiness beyond all words was just to be shared, not that we know, but this became my life, and I grateful I am. Sharing my passion for truth, inner wisdom and transformation. In this I found and live bliss and true abundance.

I moved from thinking that attraction is love, into compassion for myself and others, into devotion that was fulfilling me.

A master had been calling me in magical ways … a love affair beyond it all. … To live in union with the whole. Today I call this living in bliss.

To live from our heart is one of the biggest gift we can give to ourselves, and to the world today. . There, true abundance is found, and it is the alchemy in our life. It is important in all our areas in life. To be successful with this connection gives true value. In true relating to being love, respect and awareness. A deep gift as a parent, fellow traveler.

Love as the true teacher, no matter how hurt you may feel when someone you love leaves you, It is the other side of letting Someone you love the freedom to go…. Embracing the pain, burning in it and you will be transformed into higher levels of you being. I know by experience some really tuff ones. They always lead us into next love affair, on a higher plane. Life always wants to polish and being us into higher or clearer consciousness. So let people you love go free … in life and into the beyond. It is only our fear and unawareness that makes us controlling. Love and embrace your pain, then it will melt, heal and transform you.

It was my mothers death when I was young that made me later to start looking within. Because I loved her so deeply, I had no other choice than to feel the pain and all helplessness. It took me through all levels of pain, fairing and back into deep healing love. There peace was found. We come and we go… and to accept what we can't change is to live a big love affair to ourself and life.

If you love your partner, share it. If you have passion for your working situation, expand in it. If you don't have passion in your life see where you can find it… Your heart is the door.

If you can live love in all areas in your life – to feel at peace, with your partner … your work … your friends … your body,… yourself, your creativity and your children … to bring presence and awareness into this ever changing world. To bring awareness and truth into each and every part. To be here now ... to accept and start walking in a direction where the flow of love is for you.

Trust love and life will be a blissful adventure. Share it... live it...

In Short My Experience

I needed to step over on to my own side, and to love me, before I could really love anyone else. It is the foundation for all in my life, health and wealth. Love as medicine for all. It is the foundation together with awareness. Living from the hearts silent true wisdom. Is a life in abundance and bliss for me.

To live in pure acceptance of what is, is to stop all inner wars, all fighting, all power trips ... is to live in harmony with what is ...

Love is the healer and strongest power in the world, living in you. When **you love, no one can take it away from you.**

Meditation and Awareness Practice

Just be alive, living wisely in pure acceptance of what is, no judging. Listen to your heart and weight a love and commitment letter to your self. .

'Except man, nobody lies. A rosebush cannot lie. It has to produce roses; it cannot produce marigolds; it cannot deceive. It is not possible for it to be otherwise than it is. Except man, the whole existence lives in truth. Truth is the religion of the whole existence except man. And the moment a man also decides to become part of existence, truth becomes his religion'. — Osho

Chapter 5

Living in a yes!

Just jump into the river of life , start living it Say Yes!... Life is carrying you, holding your hand, knowing what you need ... It is high time to celebrate ... all is included here ...

Say yes to life, it has its own wisdom,
everything else will make you suffer.
Living in a yes to life! The door to bliss!
Life is always here and now for you ...
Being the centre person in your own life ... you are already
here, in the river of life ... start living and be an open part of
it ... Life is carrying you, holding your hand, knowing what
you need ... It is high time to celebrate ... all is included ...
It is a magical experience including all healing
and polishing on our way home.

Living in a yes! Stop fighting what is and the door to bliss opens ...

Bliss is 'living in endless abundance'
True wealth starts with a true melting and yes to life ...

'Courage is a love affair with
the unknown …' — Osho

Say yes to life … it wants you here! Stop fighting it, to find the way to living in bliss, and true abundance …By fighting it, you will only feel pain …

The fifth part of inner leadership is to say yes to life and your self. . We have, when trying to control life, been no sayers, trying our own ways to live. In fighting life, you will only be frustrated, feel pain and lose power. Life knows something you don't.

Heaven is already here you just have to know how to live it. And hell too is here, and you know perfectly well how to live it. It is only a question of bringing awareness and change your perspective, your approach towards life, to move from a fighting and not trusting it ..into trust and celebrating in it.What relationship so you have with lifetime self? Do you trust it or are you in conflict…?

Once I thought it was only trying to hurt me. Now I know it here for me, happing for all my best .. so is it for all of us. We just need to understand that truth.

To move with life, to have a feeling of intuition. You don't 'know' but your inner self has a feeling. To move from fighting life into trusting and saying yes is one of the most important steps to leading yourself in life. To fight life is to be in constant pain. If you have a desire and you can do something, do it… if you can't do anything or change... just let it go. Only painful experiences will come out of that. Your true abundance is beyond control and fighting. Intuition is the voice of inner truth. To follow that. To understand the we are invited here to live this life. It is like an all-inclusive charter trip. It wants us here. The question is, do we want us here? This gift is an adventure, to trust all the possibilities that come with it.

It is like jumping into a river. You can float with it, relax into it, or you can start swimming with it. Both are possible. To relax into its invisible power and wisdom ... or to see that you have the power to swim in a direction you like ... fighting And trying to control it make you frustrated and stressful.

If you swim upwards, you will have a heavy load on your shoulders, fighting and only using your energy in fighting its current and not for your life purpose.

From the now moment when I fell on the floor, asking for help, my life started to change ... into the magic of it all ... opening up, turning the pain into ease with truth, love and aliveness ...

I dropped the old and the new was coming.

Align yourself with life ... it is here for you. Effortlessly live with it ...

Live in a yes and your whole life will change ... trust will grow ... and you will find that all you ever need is coming to you. Imagine a river that flows ... trust the invisible power in it ... it has its own invisible power and direction towards the ocean ... to become one with the whole ... To live in acceptance ... fighting life will only bring you into pain, frustration and into a losing battle. Life is not a problem to be solved, it is a mystery to be lived and to be trusted.

In this I don't say you don't need to co work with life. In being free you can respond from a present now moment....

We are always in the right place at the right time. So relax and be calm, flow with life. Today I see this as having self-confidence and as receiving true abundance.

Today I know that this is included in the magic of life. I see this as living in bliss ... Life is yours to step into and wake up in ...

There is no separation between you and life ... when you don't fight the wisdom of life ... it always guides you in a higher direction ... one day without your body.

In my life experience ...

Living in a yes and it all expands perfectly.

For me to say yes in an aware conscious way was the biggest challenge. I had been so shy in my old way of living now to start step out and be responsible and aware was quite something else. But so freeing. To know that you / me and the divine is of highest order..

Life is not a serious affair, it is a joyous, loving, adventurous affair. Life took me by my hand and guided. Before I was too serious with everything, living in fear and control. Now my life for soon 40 years or so, has been so abundant and blissful. To share from my open heart, in connection with the whole, trusting the divine wisdom is one of the biggest gifts for me. To see and know that life really wants me here … Say yes, and life happens. Business, love affairs, living situation.. to follow the flow of it all.

I did or do not have any vision… life it self maybe have..My trust is in the energy.

After years of being in a melting process, I started to celebrate more and more, relaxing more, presence, loving myself and others in transforming meditations. In the presence of a master, Osho. Sitting silent, dancing and living in his presence. Pure reflections of my inner self. To understand that life is not a problem to be solved, it is a mystery to be lived … and enjoyed. Osho often reminded us all about that, and to say yes. It took some time for me to understand that. Osho left his body. Even if that was a big shift, his presence never left. And for me it was even more clear he was a light, or a true presence, and made a connection to the divine energy within me. He had always been, but now it was clearer than ever.

But one day it changed, and I was invited to start sharing. Back in Sweden where I have my roots.Coming back to Sweden and Scandinavia …Life started to guide me.little did I know. I was invited to start to work with a Norwegian leadership consultant, to work with the board of an Norwegian department store. Also was asked to start running 'meet yourself' groups in a group place Sweden. It all started to come to me. Nothing I ever thought of.. to be a group leader. Or to creat processes. But life told me differently. This gifts to practice sharing. I was also starting running groups at the Swedish Osho centre at the time.

It all just took of.

After some years I was part of starting up one of the most successful group places in Sweden, Bara Vara. It has transformed and still is transforming so many individuals in Sweden. I created the 'the door opening process', to open the door to your inner self. It became a big success and soon the groups were filling up … I think I had around two groups a month. Filled with bliss and the great fullness life is. I feel like I was sitting in group room more or less for years. Loving it.

Thousands of hearts were and are transformed through all this.

But even if so life moves and changes happens. If not on the working scene, so it happens on the love scene. I am married today to my inner truth and can't be married in any other way. But love stories happen.. and friendship in that, one big break was to fall in love and having the opportunity to be in Hawaii for some time..at a big beautiful beach in Kauai. Loved it but life moved me back to Stockholm.

It became a success. I today still lead groups like 'coming home, 'the Leap', and more and more Bliss retreats.

I feel so blessed for it all.

As magic as it all is, life took my hand and I was guided beyond my own understanding into new ways of working, living and sharing … I can't today understand how it all became possible since I did not have any vision in my mind … I had always been so shy. But now I just followed … since Osho also guided me from within as I felt it.

Life was there and is always here with us. I practiced saying yes … and still am. Now, 30 years later, and after thousands of people passing by In my life. Transforming and experiencing there inner self. them self. All just happening for me. It does fir all of us.

To live in union within as without. Life has become a meditation for me I did not have a vision.. but if you have start to see why you need to say yes to today in that direction.

All in life happens for us. When surrender happened, it all started to flow in the direction it is supposed to. I could start seeing and becoming aware of it all unfolding and happening. Now, many years later, so much bliss and true abundance has come into my life …

To become aware of the facts, life has a plan for us all.

To live in tune with your inner truth and life, you can become aware that it all comes and goes, as it is supposed to. It has all happened, coming and going in perfect celebration, mostly in loving acceptance.

All has been part of my life journey, guiding me deeper and deeper into trusting what is. All supporting me to let go and rise … life is always here for us … even in challenging times. Now, when we all share this challenging time … when turning within and trusting what is and standing on your own side … it all becomes possible for a new direction. We can't know if it is a misfortune or a blessing. We can just live in trust with what is. …

Today, I call this living in alignment ... in an alignment that brings true abundance endlessly ...

Life is not a serious affair, it is an abundant adventure ... to say yes and to enjoy the journey. To experience life in all possible ways. To experience all polarities good-bad, bitter-sweet, dark-light, summer-winter. Allow yourself to experience it all. Don't be afraid ... the more you experience, the more abundant you will feel ... bliss will be in your nature. Live and being total in all. From active to receptive happenings...

Life always wants the best for you and takes you to higher and higher experiences ... if you allow it ... if you fight it and don't trust, you may find yourself running around in circles, even needing deeper experiences before trust enters ...

Fighting life gives you pain ... letting go into the dance if it is in trust, you can start enjoying it ... and your response is easy ... present ... aware and in harmony with the whole.

Fighting life is when we believe in our minds thoughts instead of moving deeper into trust and truth here and now.

Be aware if your thought they are holding on to the old.

The freedom that we think we get from saying 'no' to others is a very childish and a very unaware kind of freedom. The opposite is true. It is good when you are seven years old or a teenager ... practicing putting up your own borders, but in a spiritual sense and awakening, it is not useful at all. It does not give you freedom. You are focused on the other, not on yourself, not on trusting life and being alive. The truth is, it is only stopping you from living free. You get caught up in thinking you need to put limits on others, and this whole life becomes a no-saying, then you have stopped growing. Living in yes is freedom and life affirming ...

By taking your life into your own hands, with no one to blame, you become a free living human being. This is a radical responsibility. The rebellious spirit of the heart and truth. If you don't become free within yourself, your life does not have the quality of adventure, of a search, of enquiry, you will remain same again and again. You will remain thirsty. You will remain unreleased ... Accept the situation you are in. It must be the right situation for you; that's why you are in it. Existence cares for you. It is given to you, not without any reason. Nothing is accidental.

Whatsoever is your need, it is given to you. Existence cares, it wants the best for you.

Our mind needs to be open to receiving the adventure of life.
Be a co-designer of your own life ... do not fight your life adventure.

In Short My Experience

Living in a yes, brings so much joy and blessings... Trust grows and to be alive becomes an adventure and a pure blessing. To become aware that life happens for us... I relax.

I call this today following the path of love in true acceptance. In this way true health and wealth is possible, blissful living as result.

Meditation and Awareness Practice

Like in nature, say yes to the silent power within …
Write a love letter to life …

'"Bliss" is the only criterion for life.
If your life is not blissful then
know you are moving wrong.
Suffering is the criterion of being wrong
and bliss is the criterion of being right
— there are no other criteria'.
— Osho, The Inner Journey

Chapter 6

Your creativity and potential are divine!

To allow you to unfold in your own inner creativity and potential
… the Bambu process, is to open the seed, grow roots and the
rest will flower by itself … standing in your own new shoes,
witnessing, innocently, bliss and true abundance unfolding …
Trust your inner potential and creativity
to be expressed, it is divine!
To explore the divine joy and creativity within you.
Witness your inner uniqueness to come through …

To allow you to unfold in your own potential … the
Bambu process, is to grow deep roots and then the rest
will happen by itself … standing in your own new shoes,
witnessing, innocently, bliss and abundance unfolding …

Trust your inner potential and creativity. It is innocent and divine!

Witness your own expression and expansion in
life, and receive it with an open heart …

Bliss 'living in endless abundance'
True wealth starts within your own source … share it …

'The life yet to come is far more important than the life behind you'.

Your inner potential is the divine expression in you … let it liberate you … witness it passing through you.

Like a seed becomes the flower … so also is your potential …

The sixth part in this inner leadership is to understand that our inner potential and creativity is divine and unique … is to live and share our own authenticity. To expand in that ever expanding and flowering energy, unique and divine, like an inner silent voice that longs to be expressed. Like a seed that is opening up and starting to grow. What potential are you hiding within your self?

Since I once I was useless, the experience in life to witness both Successfully group transforming processes and book writing… coming from within… nowhere else. We are all sitting on a treasure box.

To witness your inner potential is to trust it, to allow it to be expressed and in that your self- confidence grows.

Imagine a flower or butterfly coming out of its old form, witnessing you coming out of your own form. To open up yourself to yourself … trusting why is within that loves to be expressed. From seed to flower … to allow yourself to expand and express … truth unfolding is to be in a love affair with life and the beyond.

Never fear or hold on to your inner potential, it is divine. Stop judging your inner longing, wanting to be expressed in creative ways ... Let yourself blossom, let light surround and support you. It is like a seed when it cracks open, from which a new life, a unique flower, starts to grow.

It is the same with you ... and all of us. You can be identified with it, without being attached. You can flower freely.

In my life ... after approximately seven years of deepening within my self, meditating, e

Bringing light into all inner corners. Sitting and meeting Osho, growing in trust rising in awareness, life took my hand and guided me to share. It was like a push from within... an inner guidance to move out into the world. I feel blessed today that I was and is guided this way... even if I was trying to fight at first Since it was so nice to be surrounded by fellow travelers this way.

Life is continuing to push or guide me and us all. To get the parts of female receptiveness, and the make active parts together ... to bring the feeling of receptiveness into my mind and to express it. A challenge and a beautiful experience.

Your potential knows. Let it unfold and be expressed. You are the witnessing of it. Effortlessly ... abundant and blissful. Live and be the true version of you.

In my life experience ...

The inner potential knows something I don't ... Trust the inner longing...

I had no ideas about becoming a group leader, but that happened. Being asked to share and run groups it was easy to say yes to that. Even if my shyness needed to go. To run and later create transformative group processes … the group leading happened as gifts from without … I was scared as crazy at first … but slowly, slowly it worked it self out for me.

Book writing comes from an another energy. Here I needed to be acting by self. It was not like I was asked .. I was having a feeling of being pregnant. Like an inner calling. It was really like being pregnant with something that needed to be expressed. Our inner potential and energy is the divine hiding within to be expressed. It is consciousness itself. Also here I was totally vulnerable to put words on my experiences. But to follow what is, is to be true.

I have always been sharing from an emotional intuitive and receptive energy. To put words on to that not so easy for me. But I have learned so much from my inner that I can only bow down to that.

So never fight your inner…if making music, painting, dancing, creating in wood or anything else … go for it.. bring it into manifestation… enjoy the witnessing of it.

Book writing … putting words to my experiences … what a challenge … sharing in a new way. My first book, *New Life Vision: The Art of Living* (only in Swedish), took me six years to write. And it is now some years since it came out.

To write has given me a new witnessing awareness. I love it even if it is mainly happen four o'clock in the morning, then the channel is open.

A challenge, very challenging and beautiful. So fulfilling … a feeling of wholeness and being in ones with creation. Big words but this is how it feels. To be heal. So never suppress you inner, let it be consciously be expressed, Be total, and present, enjoy.

To understand from an inner point of energy that this inner, invisible potential is unique for each and every one of us, this is bliss in my eyes. In allowing it to be expressed, true wealth and inner abundance are bound to follow. It is a way to witness the invisible as I see it. The inner calling to be expressed. Otherwise, we need to push it back and it takes a lot of energy to hold it back. In doing so, we can become sick or burned out. The inner potential is a divine expression of who we are …

It is not me doing, or you doing it is that of the beyond coming through, 'that' being lived through us.

I felt for many years before falling on the bedroom floor, a pain in my heart … I did not know what it was … like I had something inside me that was wrong. Now I know it was my divine longing, my inner divine potential calling me.

Like a rose has to fully embrace its potential and uniqueness … and when coming into full flowering, just letting go … it was the same with me to start witnessing the inner expression and it's longing, magic started to happen…beyond my own thinking. Before being identified with "not being worthy" … or "not fitting in"….

Today, I only follow what is coming from within me, which brings me joy, happiness, to allow me to live in my own authentic way, in my own rhythm. I see this as natural fulfilment. With no expectations, all these experiences are so blissful.

It is a natural living in bliss, true abundance … for all, from an egoless point of view, the inner potential is our divine source longing to expressing itself.

To be courageous and follow your inner truth without knowing. Like a seed opening up … it knows, as within so without, the journey can begin … as it did for me when falling on the floor one morning … there and then the shell was opening … to surrender to what is … truth … loving, living it! And trusting that … life knows … the potential knows.

Always listen to your inner self, it knows … and it wants to be expressed … to be the witnessing of the potential … is to be free … celebrate it when it happens, be grateful but don't get identified … identification makes us stop growing.

To allow your inner potential to enjoy life itself with overflowing joy … Close your eyes and meditate, let the truth come surface and you will know.

Stepping into witnessing your inner alive creativity to be expressed in pure abundance. You can't be identified … just very grateful and thankful to your inner self for the gift it is bringing … pure abundance …

To work with what you love. And have passion for. Making your work into a love affair. Bringing your authentic quality into it. … dance, paint, write, play music sing … All inner potential is divine!

We are all carrying a masterpiece, and superpower, hidden within. Allowing your creativity to be a meditation in expression and expansion … Courage and creativity go together … To, dance, sing, paint, and live is to let go … into not knowing. Your inner divine knows … It all comes from a place within you where you can't think about it …

Your inner potential is endlessly abundant … like a rose bush that continues giving and giving its flowers … there is nowhere to go, there is just being here and celebrating …

Your potential is aligned with the whole universal wisdom and will, no separation exists … Creativity is like a divine 'pregnancy'.

All ideas and superpower are coming from within. Release, trust and witness …

Dance, sing, play music, paint, write … allow your inner to be released. Bring this quality into your life when being with family, friends, on your morning walk, to your work …

sing in the car … release your soul and spirit … from where is it coming and where is it going? …

To allow, be alive …

To expand and express

To trust your own uniqueness

In Short My Experience

The inner potential, from seed to flower .. "nothingness" into manifestation. To trust the inner and not standing in its way. Just a pure witnessing of the divine coming into flowering. My experience is to be just a watcher… in all creating. … It is not mine, it is the universal expression through me.

This I call living in a process of witnessing, allowing your inner creativity to flower … creativity as a healing meditation.

Living true abundance from within … blissful living

Meditation and Awareness Practice

What divine expression and creativity are you holding back within you? …

What Is your inner calling you to share?

What does the universe want to manifest through you?

Living and allowing your true inner potential and source, your powers will manifest in a great true way. Then fulfilment will be your experience.

'The life yet to come is far more important than the life behind you'.

Chapter 7

Relaxing into silence ... it knows!

There you will find the centre of bliss.

Presence, the invisible, the unknown, the
silence behind it all ... Just be!

Bliss and true abundance are yours to rest in Be still and know.
Resting into silence, it knows! ... Simply let go ...
and be you ... You are already it, so relax ...

Presence, the invisible, the unknown, the silence behind it all ...
Just be! Bliss and true abundance are yours to feel and rest into!

Resting into silence, it knows! ...Born to be a Buddha ...
yes.. rest like a Buddha ..live and die like a Buddha ...

Blissful living is in deep connection with stillness, silence
and the invisible source we all contain within ... to prepare
for living is one dimension ... the other is to prepare for
leaving when the time is right ... meditation is the bridge.
Bliss is 'living in endless abundance'

True wealth starts within your own source ... relax into it!
Meditation is the key.

You are what existence want you to be ... just relax'.

Be still, silent and learn to listen to wisdom deep within it, to just be ... the secret of life is showing itself in a deep letting go ...
Your inner is like an open empty sky where birds can fly ... and dark clouds can pass ... without you interfering ...

In this seventh part of this Bliss book and inner leadership, it is about to know how to relax, rest and let go. To step out of the outer circus, from all identification, to give your self a break from it all. To relax into the invisible. Your spiritual self is the truth about you. Without any concepts, resting within the conscious invisible space. The more trust you have to this the more aligned with the magic of life and the beyond you are The more blissful your life becomes.

It is to let go and take a vacation from doing and the outer world. To just be yourself, with the self....to relax. It is where you refill your batteries, can listen to truth and what is, dropping your personal goal for the goal of the whole. Leave the mind behind. for a moment.

Here we will find and get the answers we are seeking. May be silent answers, to start trusting the invisible wisdom we all contain. the greatest gift to yourself, for the whole energy system.

One day we as such will leave this life... the more you have connected to the space within you, instead of only the body, you can trust eternity. In this resting and find inner truth and harmony. Our whole immune system is affected by our energy. And the more we are living in harmony and truth, the more everything falls into the right place within us. Silently ... Just to be and to know you are this. The form, the body is like a house. This house is not who we are it is the form around who we truly are. In every breath we connect with the bigger something and eternity. You don't miss the house when leaving for going outside into fresh air. The same one day when we leave.. To learn the art of silence and non-doing, is to be, just to be. Learn to listen to the silent and stillness, to meditate, is to be ... aware, awake and to know you are not the doer ... or the house it self. Start trusting the invisible now. Breath it... feel it and To love it is the gift to you now.

All forms change. They come and go.

To start letting go of the outer and just drop within, into silence and non-doing. So for now with our body as fellow traveler, closing all your doors and windows ... just to be in solitude within for some moments every day. This is to come back home and to connect with your true essence ... When I was a child before five, I trusted life, the big something ..then I lost the connection and with that trust. Where and when did you loose trust ?

Imagine an empty sky ... no judging whatever passes on it ...

Don't waste this beautiful opportunity here and now to come home. Just give some space to be present and to melt into the grace that brought you here and continues to do its work within you ...

In my life experience …

To be, just to be is a blessing …
Trust your being…

life has such has become a meditation for me. A life in bliss, to remember my being. I thank existence for bringing this silent wisdom, and opening me into my inner self. The divine intervention is a blessing to me. From that I share… nothing else is possible.

The gaps and space between the clouds … the aliveness and the stillness. Just to allow me to be … loving me as I am … in pure presence.

Me witnessing … silence and stillness … waves passing without being attached or identified. Meditation is for me the art of being present, open, non-judging, accepting and witnessing.

The longing in my heart, the connection in my heart guiding me to Osho, a magic beyond words. I am living this love and sharing it in one way or the other silently every day of my life. This thankfulness is beyond my understanding. Giving time to step out, is to give space to step in.

Giving me months of being-ness. Meditation, sitting silently … resting into what is … together with others the presence of silence becomes stronger. A blissful experience.

We are born wise and complete. This truth is to be found within. Silently and trustingly we are embraced there. To remember this again. To stop, turn within and rest is possible for all. To connect with the inner space of silence and nothingness.

To rest in the silence beyond it all. The importance to stop, to drop out of all doings and to just be, silent and still, is fundamental.

To live and be richly inspired by the divine. To follow what is … to trust and to melt all separation. Bringing your awareness back home.

I met a master's presence … I met my presence, emptiness and total love Within me through him. … for me to live that presence, empty and the love that is when accepting what is. Together with others, was one of the most divine experience for me when we all were meeting in the evening for meditation together … the silence we all were in and moving in afterwards was for me such an experience of union and silent bliss. I wish we all could have that experience. So we could feel the oneness we all are, without doing anything.

I felt seen and loved for the first time in my life from a man sitting with closed eyes and not saying a word … even if he later spoke again …

Seeing me with my closed eyes, not saying a word. This love is the source from which sharing happens in my life … Osho's endless love is now 'my' endless love, light and blessings. I am not him. That is not what I say, but I see that what I once projected onto him … is all in me …

Keeping the projection out there, I miss the presence here and now. It makes a distance within me. Bring it home. Feeling it makes me feel the oneness we all are, beyond all mind and understanding.

I love being devoted to that, the bigger something, and there is no separation … this is what I experience again and again, and Osho was, and still is, guiding me into this.

Meeting him was for me meeting pure emptiness, like a window to the whole existence.

A life journey beyond all gratefulness. To share inner silence in pure bliss. The most beautiful moments when being in India with Osho was when we all went into the silent evening meeting … we all had white robes … we walked into silence sitting quite close at the time. Osho answered questions and gave his discourse for about 90 minutes, including music and celebration and inner guidance. As he shared in my understanding, better to listen to him talking than listening to our own mind shatter. The feeling when thousands are moving alone and together in silence in and out of the hall … some time holding someone's hand silently … just walking alone and together … the oneness and silent bliss is carried deep within me, such a blessing … that experience is ever lasting within me.

In all work I share silence in small and bigger moments … it is always a blessing. It is an important part in transforming your life into bliss and true abundance. I share from this divine overflowing space. That is all I can do.

I love sitting silently. I love Osho's transforming meditations for us modern people. I used them for years every day. They are such important tools in my group processes, as pillars for transformation, and they are so easy to download and do by yourself at home …

I share this the best way I can. Guiding individuals, in sessions, in groups, in relationships, families, companies into them self, nothing else is possible than to fennecs within … there the whole is contained.

To be alive, silent and still … to drop within your inner empty space when you can. Doing nothing but relaxing and witnessing … You don't need to be anyone … you are already …

As the poet Rumi so beautiful expressed it, 'Close your eyes, stay there and fall in love'. This is it.

To allow you to be … just to be you … and the rest will follow … conscious living … life as a meditation in total balance … allowing parts to be lived. No doing needs to be done. You simply respond to life when it comes with its gift.

My work is a meditation, it is always here and now … non-judging and totally accepting what is … In this meeting and supporting others is the transforming key. I was never a seeker but by divine blessing became more and more of a finder … that I wish to share with you all … you are the one you have been longing for … nothing is out there, it us all in here …

Your being is the pure open space of consciousness that lives within you, unaffected by external forces and circumstances.

You can only be your true self when you are present, when your thoughts are not focused on the past, future or an ego-created false identity. By connecting with your true self through presence, you access inner peace. Bliss is your nature … enjoy it. … True abundance is how life works. In this, our life is transformed …

Meditation is to stop and be present, non-judging, not being identified with mind, or parts … allowing the energy to flow freely, seeing it, accepting what is … not only looking into the emptiness within, but resting there, enjoying it, being embraced by it, with no desire to fill it, to witness what is. To understand that all life has its source within, and all creativity and successes are coming from this inner silent truth. It is already full. It is your source of abundance. It looks empty because you don't have the understanding or awareness of it ... When you see it through the mind, you lose the connection. That is the way of misunderstanding ... If you put the mind aside and look into your emptiness... not fearing it.. Just feeling it and being it.

I was not a seeker from a spiritual aspect but I did become a finder in my heart and being.

It is such tremendous beauty, it is divine, it is overflowing with joy. Nothing else is needed. Living in silent bliss. It has its own wisdom.

As Lau Tzu once explained,

'Sitting silently, doing nothing, the grass grows by itself'.

You can't do silence ... you can just remove or step out of the way ... like the sky is always behind the clouds. Witnessing and resting in the bigger space. Allowing your focus to turn in another way than where the noise is.

To find rest, peace ... non-doing ... witnessing ... just being ... is of greatest importance. To balance yourself from all doing, just to let go. To witness and experience the truth of life.

It happens for us ...

Open your eyes to that truth ...

There is no separation, everything is perfect as it is ... so relax as deeply as possible into it all ... What wants to happen will happen ... just witness like clouds in the sky ...

Allow yourself to be still, silent and just being … resting into the silent space of magic …Let it expand.

In Short My Experience

Just to be, open and relaxed. In moments just dropping all and rest… meditation is the key. Like dying into divine nothingness, is the ultimate relaxation for me, again and again.. in this deep silent inner fulfilment is happening. Sharing silence with others are amazingly beautiful for me. In this we change the world.

Today I call this coming home … being home … shining the divine self of who we truly are. Meditation may look serious but to discover the joy and freedom in the adventure into nothingness is a pure blessing.

Meditation is like sitting on the dock of the bay … meditation is the solution …
Sit, work, love and rest …. Life becomes pure blessing. Living and dying goes together and when we can leave this life in a blissful energy after blissful life…

Sit, be, relax, all is perfectly taken cared of … Just give time to your inner self. Be still an you will know…

'The mystery never ends, it cannot end. That's why it is called a mystery, it cannot be known ever. It will never become knowledge, that's why it is called a mystery; something in it is eternally elusive. And that's the whole joy of life. The great splendor of life is that it keeps you eternally engaged, searching, exploring. Life is exploration, life is adventure'. — Osho

Trust your unique light path, and it's endless possibilities ... You are you.. respect that!

Living in endless blissfulness.

It feels totally natural for me to complete this book with *Namaste*. Namaste means 'I greet the whole within you'. Already during my time with my mother in Indonesia 1974. I learned to say and do Namaste. But it was during my years in India, more than ten years later, that I first started to understand and grasp the meaning of the words. I greet the whole and thank the divine within you. I greet the love, the peace and the truth that you are. Within you vibrates the whole universe. Start to explore and dare to meet this wholeness. Everyone has everything. No darkness can remain dark if we bring the light of awareness into it. Consciousness is all there is. Then we can see and understand. We have darkness and we have light. All polarities. When the light of consciousness is lit, everything lights up and becomes transparent. I am not filled with a lot of answers, only the experience of living a life that transformed me into love and awareness. Trusting the emptiness that is alive and contains all wisdom I will ever need. Filled with love and gratitude. For me this is divine. I wish this book to bring light and blessed change into your life.

'It is not that we are dew drops in the ocean … we are the hole ocean in a dew drop'. – Rumi

Dare to stop and starting living yourself. Respect your self and others. Trust to expand in life. Change is the only sure thing here. With a great *yes* in your divine heart, trust that life wants all good for you. Let your next step lead you into brilliance. Learn to listen to your own core of truth.

I lived in dysfunction at the beginning of my life. With a strong feeling of separation. I encountered myself and experienced that I am not my story, but that I am the consciousness and awareness beyond it – in the silence space within me, all divine is contained. We all have the capacity to transform and to experiences all tastes of this divine nectar. All is included in this blissful and truly abundant journey. That is the ultimate we all are.

Love & Namaste

Testimonials

Some feedback from participants …

'After spending a full-day group session with Premleena Lena Wettergran … I have gained a great deal. The idea of looking within has become very tangible and this new perspective. It serves as a great tool in my very demanding lifestyle. It gives me great joy to have shared this experience with my wife and some very close friends. The feeling of a shared and collective awareness has brought us all closer together'.
Ben, 41 / married with 2 kids. Creative Director of a global luxury brand

'It's overwhelming so much power there is within me … I have been afraid and have said no to myself my whole life … had panic attacks and was living in control, with myself and others … getting very angry when life, or my partner, kids, business associates were not doing or living my way … now I feel I can more and more relax and trust … I love my inner connection and my being … I don't react, I can act with awareness … I feel real love for the first time in my adult life … sooo grateful'.
Caroline, 39/ businesswoman … with her own business … 2 kids and a loving husband …

'Deep thank you for bringing awareness into my life … Have been longing for this long for a long time … Wish all people to get this support … I can share more and more with my own clients … understanding our human nature … It is really all about loving acceptance and awareness. The way Premleena shares this is just so natural and easy … like no obstacles or threats in opening up … I had a lot of that in me before we met … Only Blessings from me …'
Camilla, 50/ woman bodyworker, chiropractor

'I have been seeing Premleena for private sessions for over a year, and this was my first experience in a group. Although this group was comprised of close friends and family, my experience was beyond what I could have imagined. The shared awareness opened a channel of energy for me that I can only describe as a completely new perspective. I am truly grateful for the insightfulness I continue to gain, and the group session has contributed another dynamic tool for me and my family to grow and connect on our journey. Imagine a world that could share energy this way … what a blessing that would be'.
Natasa, 39/ woman with a husband and 2 kids

'I was invited by a dear friend of mine to spend a whole day with Premleena. We were a small group of five, some that I already knew and others I met for the first time.
I did not know what to expect from the day, and I had only heard of Premleena through my friend who invited me.
I was curious and also a little bit nervous, but as soon as we arrived to the beautiful house where Premleena greeted us, I immediately felt very safe.

It was an absolutely magical day, with so many feelings passing through.

I laugh, I cried, I shared feelings and thoughts with others, I danced in the sunlight, and I reflected in silence.

I spent time with a part of me that I have neglected.

I am so grateful and happy for what I experienced, and I will carry that day with me forever'.

Anna, 42/woman yoga teacher

'I feel so fulfilled in my life … I just need to share with you. I have finally become free of mind …'

I did two groups with Premleena a long time ago … Door opener 1, and 2 … They created a new foundation and platform in my life …

They started a transformation that has slowly been manifesting in my life … in perfect speed and order … I can say from my heart, I bow down to you for the courage of standing there for all of us … I love you for that … I love me for the courage of listening to my inner pain and not being satisfied with the way things where … Now I simply love myself and life for the perfection of it all. Big hug.

Erik, 49

'It was 1970 when colour tv came. From black and white … into a world filled with colors.

The year 2019 was when Premleena came into my life. She turned me into opening up to my inner self, bought my life into an alive transformation and awakening. My life has since then, piece by piece, become abundant, richer with colours in all areas of my life. Also, the darkness within me has been brought into the light, where the parts have become more and more interesting, instead of scary, as it was very much before I met her. The big shift for me was the day I could see that all was within me. I was 'jealous of myself' in my own life. So strange but true. The life change was obvious. Premleena, is fantastic – challenging, questioning, inspiring, supportive in the process of growing in awareness, presence and love. In all parts of life and issues. She is the most loving human being I have ever met in my life.

I feel so much gratefulness that she entered my life. She has the capacity power, awareness skill, to put light onto the parts that were and are not visible for me. She helped me find the treasures within me. I think that awareness is all that matters for me in life today … after a successful career, a marriage that broke, two beautiful, alive kids, a house and a stable with horses, a life in the country. A new awareness about myself … my thoughts, my feelings and the present space beyond that.

Premleena, thank you for being you, for sharing all you share so generously, lovingly, all wisdom and that you included me in that. It is pure magic … Deep, deep gratitude on my side.

Kattis/30 on the way to 40 …

One of my clients who stopped running away from herself … and turned within almost 20 years ago … 'I had never spent an hour in therapy the day I ended up in a group process with Premleena. Not because I didn't need it. It was because I was so filled with shame, and therapy was the ultimate proof of my 'incapability', being a victim. I was a 'professional' in running away from myself. I was a workaholic, shopaholic, party princess, going to the gym as much as possible and drinking far, far too much. Everything you can put words to … I had no self-awareness at all …

Getting my inner puzzle together was impossible … In other people's eyes, I was a very 'successful' young beautiful woman. Very competent, True in the world of money, having an impressive job, knowing all and everyone in the ' important' world … and had a very rich social life. On the inside, in my inner world it was another story … Even if I was young, I often thought

… 'is this really all there is in life ?' 'What is the point of it all … ?' Pain was knocking from within without me wanting to feel it …

I met a friend of mine just coming back from one of these group experiences … it was just a coincidence … She was shining, a beaming light … I booked a group after that … I also wanted to be a light like that … even if my self-esteem was low. As the run-away person I was, I had never read information about the process. I thought it was a kind of a spa … with walks in nature … Finally, when going there, Premleena received me with so much wisdom, patience, humour, presence and love. All I longed for … It was a sure door opener to my inner self, meeting pain, abandonment and sorrow.

I didn't know I was also, behind all this, carrying all my answers, inner knowing and loving potential, something I never thought possible. I was so unaware and needed keys to my inner self. I respect Premleena and her work very much, and all the groups I have been participating in. I feel so much gratefulness also to myself for daring to look within … And if I could wish for something, I would wish all people could experience the same feeling as I, spending a few days together with her. Believe me, if I dared, you can dare …

With tons of love and gratefulness …

Charlotta … 48 years old and working as a happy professional project organizer for celebrities …

Author bio

Lena Premleena Wettergran

The author of *Blissful living : A Guide to Transform Your Life NOW!*

She is a well known coach and group leader in Sweden, since thirty five years. Being an Osho counseling therapist, a reiki healing master since 1986. Since then she help individuals, leaders, teams and couples. All with a longing to grow into more awareness and love. To go from pain, stress and a feeling of being disconnected… stressed out, not belonging or being wrong. She knows because she was once there her self. Working hard striving and running fast for something she didn't know what it was… until one morning a full stop happened… Transformation started to happen, she started to move from pain into a healing wise heart, This opened the depth of a healing and wisdom beyond she was aware of. In this pure presence she started to trust her self and life. .

Now she is having the experience of helping thousands of people to come home in there own energy, , finding peace and deeper meaning in life, daring to trust and live there own truth in life.. to follow the wisdom of there hearts. This is what many many people todays needs to find, an inner connection and bliss. ,.. From fearing life into saying yes…

Just a turn within and little bit of awareness is all that is needed...

She offers retreats, sessions, trainings, talks and group processes that provide healing for body mind and soul... she meets individuals, couples, leaders, companies, sports teams and organisations.These sessions and group retreats bring you home to your own inner silent wisdom and knowing. Transformation is possible for all and in all areas of life. It affect your health, wealth, way of loving and leading your self and others. As within so without.

When stepping out of the old, magic really start to happens ... Blissful living is the magic of life itself. The biggest gift you can give to yourself. Invest and transform your life now.

Www.premleena.se/com

www.ingramcontent.com/pod-product-compliance
Lightning Source LLC
Chambersburg PA
CBHW032101020426
42335CB00011B/450